Coping with advanced cancer

This booklet aims to help people who have been told their cancer has spread or come back. It is also for their relatives and friends. The booklet discusses common concerns and problems, and advises on how to cope with them.

Not all the information will apply to you, and you may find that the booklet talks about things that do not affect you or that you do not want to read about. The list of contents will help you to identify the sections that you want to read and feel would be most helpful to you.

You may have been told that it is not possible to cure your cancer. While no one can predict for certain what will happen to a particular person, your doctors will have said this on the basis of the evidence and their experience. It may be possible, although it is rare, for an advanced cancer to be cured. Treatment can usually be given which will help to control the cancer and prolong life, perhaps for a number of years, although sometimes just for a number of months. For some people, it may not be possible to treat the cancer itself. However, treatment can be given to control symptoms, such as pain.

This booklet looks at the concerns that people with advanced cancer often have. It discusses the many and varied emotions and feelings that you may face at this time. It also has information about practical concerns, such as the support that may be available to you. We hope that this booklet will help you to be able to live with your cancer, in the way that is best for you.

If you find this booklet helpful, you can pass it on to family and friends, who may want information so they can support you.

Throughout this booklet you will find quotations from people with advanced cancer. We thank all those people who have shared their feelings and experiences with us.

Contents

My cancer has come back

Learning that your cancer has spread, or come back, may be even more devastating than hearing for the first time that you have cancer. It may be hard to take it in – your thoughts may be in complete turmoil, or your mind may go blank. This shock and disbelief can give way to strong – often overwhelming – emotions.

'I don't remember the journey home. It was like a film without any soundtrack – a jumbled mass of meaningless images.'

People often have a sense of loss, or feelings of failure. You had hoped that you were cured and now find your cancer has come back despite your efforts to overcome it. You may find yourself tearful and depressed for some time. Some people are stunned and resentful to see life going on as normal around them when their own world is in such turmoil.

Fear

Many people are afraid. You may be afraid of the illness itself; the treatment; the effect it may have on your family; symptoms such as pain; or dying.

Anger

You may feel very angry – with yourself, or with the doctors and nurses, for giving you bad news. You may be angry at fate, feeling that it is so unfair that this should have happened. You may be resentful and frustrated that your immediate plans will be disrupted with tests and treatment, and that your long-term plans have suddenly become uncertain.

Looking ahead

Small shocks may distress you: tiny decisions like 'Is it worth paying my subscription this year? – I may not be here long' or 'I'd love to buy some new clothes – but will I ever get to wear them?'

Different people have different emotions. Living with the uncertainty that comes with the spread or recurrence of cancer is likely to be physically and emotionally demanding. If you had hoped that your cancer was cured, it can be very hard to have to make decisions about treatment again, about what to tell your family, friends and people at work, and about what adjustments to make to your home life. There are many sources of help and some of these are listed at the back of this booklet.

'I rarely cried in the early days with the condition but since the secondary sites were confirmed I find I cry more readily, and the release of emotion helps enormously because I get very pent-up.'

What you can do

- Be aware of the emotions you are feeling. It is natural and normal to feel a whole range of powerful emotions when your life is suddenly turned upside-down by illness. There are many ways you can get help to enable you to work through and deal with your emotions.

- If you can, find someone you can talk to about how you are feeling – perhaps a family member or friend, a nurse or other carer, or a religious or spiritual leader. If you feel uncomfortable talking about these things with someone you know, you may find that you would prefer to join a support group, or to see a counsellor (see pages 46–52)

- Remind yourself of ways in which you have dealt with other difficult situations in the past. Remember the strengths you had then, and see if you can use them again now.

Services such as Cancerbackup can be helpful in giving support and information at this time.

Deciding about your treatment

Some people are happy to have whatever treatment their doctor recommends, but others like to know as much as possible before starting any course of treatment.

There are several different types of treatment that may be appropriate, depending on your type of cancer and where it is in the body. Surgery, radiotherapy, chemotherapy, hormonal therapies, biological therapies, or a combination of treatments may be offered. Often, treatment will be aimed at relieving symptoms and improving your quality of life. This is sometimes called palliative care or supportive care.

Talking about treatment options

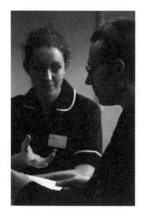

It is usually possible to take a bit of time to think about the treatment options, and discuss them with the people closest to you and the doctors and nurses looking after you. Your oncologist (cancer specialist) is the best source of accurate medical information. In some hospitals, specialist nurses are available to talk over all the possible benefits and side effects of treatment, and whether you want to have further treatment or not.

Remember that the treatment is designed to be for your benefit. It is important that you make the decision that feels right for you about which treatment, if any, you are prepared to have; even if your family or doctors may recommend otherwise.

It is often difficult to remember the questions you want to ask your doctor. It may help you to make a list before your next appointment. Some people find it helpful to record the discussion with the doctor, or take a friend or family member with them. As well as giving support, they may be able to take notes for you, or remind you of any questions that you want to ask. Tapes can also be helpful for family and friends to listen to, so that you do not have to repeat information again and again if they also have questions.

Some questions you could ask your specialist

- What are my treatment options?
- Is this treatment aimed at curing the cancer, helping me to live longer or dealing with my symptoms?
- What benefits should I expect from the treatment?
- Are there any side effects? Are they temporary or permanent?
- Will I have to change my diet?
- Will the cancer or treatment affect my sex life?
- Will I need time off work?
- Will I need to stay in hospital and, if so, for how long?
- If treatments are given as an outpatient, how long will each one take and how many will I need?
- Should somebody take me to and from hospital, or will I be able to drive or travel by myself?
- What can I do to help myself?

Who can give information?

You may find it difficult to collect your thoughts in a busy out-patients clinic, and many questions are likely to come up between your hospital appointments or visits to the doctor. The nurses at our cancer support service can discuss your situation and give you information and emotional support. Both patients and their relatives sometimes find it helpful to talk to someone they do not know, and who is not emotionally involved in their situation.

Symptom control

Your doctor may suggest that there is no further treatment that can be given to control your cancer. This does not mean that 'nothing more can be done', but instead that the aim of treatment is changing. Rather than trying to shrink the cancer, the aim will now be to ease troublesome or distressing symptoms. This will make sure that you are comfortable and will give you the best possible quality of life.

No treatment

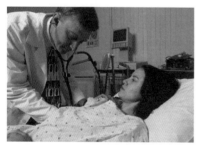

If you decide against any treatment, the hospital may suggest that you still come in for regular check-ups. Instead, you may be discharged to the care of your GP. They will probably also want to see you regularly, to check how you are getting on and to have a chance to recommend medicines which may help you, and ways of making you more comfortable.

Complementary and alternative therapies

Some people wonder whether complementary or alternative therapies can help them when they are told that their cancer cannot be cured. We can send you a booklet about complementary therapies and cancer. Although complementary therapies cannot cure cancer, they can sometimes help to reduce symptoms, and can give a sense of well-being, which can be helpful in coping with advanced cancer (see pages 21–22).

You may see alternative therapies advertised: these cannot cure cancer. They can also be harmful to some people. It is important to discuss with your doctor any therapy you are thinking of trying.

Research – clinical trials

Research into new ways of treating advanced cancer and controlling symptoms is going on all the time. Current treatments can be helpful for many people with advanced cancer, but may cause unpleasant side effects.

Cancer doctors (oncologists) are continually looking for better ways of treating cancer and controlling symptoms, and they do this by using clinical trials. Any new drug that is developed will go through trials to check that it is safe to give and is effective.

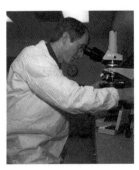

If early research suggests that a new treatment or medicine might be more effective than the standard treatment, doctors will carry out trials to compare the new treatment with the best ones currently available. Several hospitals around the country often take part in these trials. Called controlled clinical trials, they are the only way of scientifically testing a new treatment. Until new treatments have been tested scientifically in this way, it is impossible for doctors to know which treatment is best for their patients. Just because something is new, it does not mean that it is better than the treatment that already exists. Your doctor may suggest to you that you consider taking part in trials to test an experimental treatment, or to compare a newer treatment with the standard one.

Giving consent

Your doctor must have your **informed consent** before entering you into any clinical trial. This means that you know what the trial is about, you understand why it is being done and why you have been invited to take part, and that the treatment has been discussed with you.

Even after agreeing to take part in a trial, you can still leave the trial at any stage if you change your mind. Your decision will in no way affect your doctor's attitude towards you. If you choose not to take part or withdraw from a trial, you will then have the best standard treatment rather than the new one with which it is being compared.

If you choose to take part in a trial, remember that whatever treatment you are given will have been carefully researched in preliminary studies before it is fully tested in any trial.

Newspapers, magazines, and radio and television programmes often mention new cancer treatments. Friends may also tell you about them. If you are not sure whether the treatment would be appropriate in your situation, it is helpful to discuss it with your cancer specialist, who is in the best position to advise you.

We produce a booklet, *Understanding Cancer Research Trials*, which we can send to you.

People close to you

Having cancer does not turn you into a different person. You still need love, companionship and fun. You may find that friends, family and partners become even more important to you, and are a vital source of help and support. In many cases your partner, children, parents, friends and colleagues will be waiting to take their cue from you – about how much you want to talk about your illness and the treatment.

People who have cancer sometimes feel that a great deal of responsibility lies with them, and that this is very unfair. It may seem as though you are the one who has to be strong. You may feel you have to start the difficult conversations and help friends and family members who are having problems in facing your illness, even though it is you who is ill. If you are able to talk openly, they will probably be relieved and able to respond. However, if you are unwell or feeling low, it is very difficult to take on that burden. In spite of the difficulties, you will be getting back some control if you can manage to begin these conversations.

We have a booklet called *Talking About Your Cancer*, which suggests ways that you may be able to talk to your family and friends. We can send you a copy, or you can see the information on our website: www.cancerbackup.org.uk

Serious illness does affect relationships and many people find it difficult to know how to respond. You may find that people react in unexpected ways. Some may try to deny the seriousness of the situation by being inappropriately cheerful, preventing you from showing how you feel. Others may try to avoid you rather than risk saying the wrong thing.

Some people may completely avoid discussing your illness, and others may seem unsympathetic or even abrupt and rude. Your parents or your partner may irritate you by being overprotective and trying to 'wrap you in cotton wool'. Sometimes partners try to protect each other from the truth by denying it, even though both are aware of what is really happening. If you can't talk about your situation because you become emotional, you could try writing a letter for them to read at a quiet time.

In these ways, lifelong friends and close family can sometimes feel like strangers, just at the time when you need them most. It may help to remember that everyone is shocked by bad news.

Your family and friends are also dealing with strong emotions and their initial reactions do not necessarily reflect their true feelings.

Our booklet, *Lost for Words*, is written for relatives and friends of people with cancer. It looks at some of the difficulties people may have when talking about cancer.

'No matter how much your family and friends may love you, living with an ill person is not always easy. Nobody can truly imagine your distress, and you must not blame them for that.'

Partners

Talking about your feelings with your partner can help to support you both through the sadness, worry and uncertainty. You may find that your relationship is made stronger, and you can face the challenge of your illness together, if you can both be open about your feelings. When words fail you, or seem inadequate for a particular moment, just being together, or having a hug, can say as much – and sometimes more – than words.

There may be times when you do not get on well together. Just at the time when you need each other most, the stresses of an uncertain future, or the difficulties and side effects of treatment, can put a strain on your relationship. You may find that problems are harder to resolve because you feel you have less time to consider compromises.

Anger can be a common problem for both yourself and your partner. It may help to relieve the stress if you give yourselves short breaks from each other, to think more calmly and 'recharge your emotional batteries'. Sometimes talking to someone else can help. Perhaps a friend or relative, or someone completely outside your situation, like a counsellor. If this seems a sensible idea, it may be best to discuss it with your partner first, so they do not feel excluded, or that they have failed you.

Your sex life

There is no medical reason to stop having sex because you have cancer. Cancer is not catching, and sex of any sort will not make your cancer worse. In fact, a sexually loving relationship can generate warmth, comfort and a sense of well-being that can be very supportive.

You may find that your illness has no effect on your sex life. On the other hand, you may find that you cannot or do not want to have sex in the ways you did before you were ill. This may be because of the physical effects of the treatment or the disease; for example, because you feel too tired or sick, or because your worries make it difficult to feel enthusiastic about sex. It may be that the treatment (for example, surgery) has changed your appearance, which can make you feel self-conscious and inhibited about sex.

Your partner may also have concerns about your illness and its effect on your physical relationship; perhaps a fear of hurting you while making love. But you need not deny your sexual needs and desires. There are many ways of sharing love and finding satisfaction.

If you can be honest and open with your partner, you can help each other to find ways of expressing your love for each other. Intercourse is not the only kind of physically satisfying sex. Slow, sensual touching, stroking and kissing bring as much, and sometimes more, enjoyment. Cuddles and affectionate kisses can also show how much you care for someone, even if you don't feel like having sex.

You do not need to feel guilty or embarrassed to ask for professional advice if you are having sexual problems. People with cancer have as much right to an active and satisfying sex life as anyone else. Your doctor or nurse may be able to advise you directly, or they can refer you and/or your partner for specialist counselling if you think that would be helpful.

We have a booklet, *Sexuality and Cancer*, which discusses these issues in more detail.

Children

It is never easy, and can be very painful, to talk to your children or grandchildren about cancer. It is probably best to talk honestly with them and to tell them that your cancer has come back or spread.

Even very young children will sense when something serious is going on. However much you want to protect your children, if you pretend to them that everything is fine, they will feel that they have to keep their worries to themselves, and their fears may be far worse than the reality. They may feel isolated and excluded and not able to tell you how sad and upset they are.

Children may feel that they are in some way responsible for a parent's or grandparent's illness, and if you can discuss your cancer with them, you can reassure them that they are not.

How and what you tell your children will depend on their age and how much they can understand. It may be a good idea to choose a time to tell them when you, your partner, close friends or relatives can all be together, so that the children will know that there are other adults they can share their feelings with, and who will support them.

There is probably no need to go into too much medical detail. You can just explain simply about your illness, and the treatment you are having. It might be helpful to warn your children about how they may be affected – for example, that there will be days when you will feel too ill or tired to be able to play with them or join in their activities. If you have to go back into hospital, you can tell them how often you would like them to visit you and that they can write or telephone. If you talk a bit about your feelings, this may help them to express theirs.

We have a booklet called *Talking to Children About Cancer*, which may be helpful.

Children can react in many different ways to your illness, and some of these may be hard to deal with. For example, they may start to behave badly to cover up their feelings of insecurity. They may withdraw from you for fear of being hurt, or become very clingy because they are anxious that something might happen to you when they are not there. They may be angry and resentful that you are not able to do things with them in the way you used to.

Children will need lots of reassurance that your illness makes no difference to your love for them. They will also need reassurance on practical things – who will take and fetch them from school, for example, if you are not well enough to do so. It will help them if, as far as possible, their routines are not disturbed and their daily lives continue as normally as you can manage.

Teenagers

Teenagers can have an especially hard time – they often experience a range of feelings in the same way that an adult does. At a time when they want more freedom, they may be asked to take on new responsibilities. It is important that they don't feel over-burdened, and that they go on with their normal lives and still get the guidance they need. If they are finding it hard to talk to you, it can be helpful to encourage them to talk to someone close who can support and listen to them, such as a grandparent, family friend, teacher or counsellor. Other people may also need to be involved in supporting children and teenagers. They could include teachers, social workers, health visitors or counsellors.

'No child – toddler or teenager – can remember your illness all the time. Young people are not capable of carrying a constant burden of grief. They must be allowed to put it down sometimes and laugh with their friends like other youngsters, without older people feeling any resentment.'

Friends and colleagues

Some friends and colleagues will feel unsure about how to talk to you and may leave it up to you to make the first move.

A quick phone call or email will show that you are keen and able to keep up social contact. You might start by saying something like: 'I'm afraid I've had some bad news about my cancer, but the treatment seems to be going well (or 'I still feel quite well') and I would like to get out and see you.'

When you contact people you can tell them whatever you want about your situation. You don't have to go into great detail.

Obviously you will not want to talk about your cancer all the time and you may rely on your friends to carry on as usual and distract you. They will probably welcome it if you can tell them what you want or need from them, whether it is help in the house; regular visits for a chat; their company on an outing; or driving you to hospital appointments.

However, there may be some friends or family members who back away from you because they feel so threatened and frightened by your illness that they cannot cope. This can be very painful. If your attempts to make contact have been rejected, you may have to try to accept that they feel this way and that there is nothing more you can do about it. However, it is important to realise that the reason they are doing this is nothing to do with you, but is due to their own difficulties in dealing with your circumstances.

If you don't want to talk

There may be times when you simply do not want to see people and just want to be on your own. Also, there may be some well-meaning friends whose reactions to your illness upset you. You can allow other people to protect you: for example, let someone else go to the door or answer the telephone. If you are in hospital you may want to limit the visitors you have. You can ask a relative or the nurses to help you with this. There is no need for you to feel that you have to see people if you do not want to or if you need time to yourself.

'I find one of the worst aspects is friends who think they are helping by offering platitudes, and also those who insist upon helping you cross the road when you don't need it, and seem to find it impossible to talk about anything else.'

If you live on your own

It may be very hard to cope and stay positive if you live alone. Even if you value your independence, being ill can make you feel very lonely and isolated.

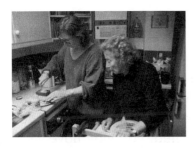 People who are close to you will want to help in any way they can. Some people will find it difficult to talk about the cancer, but would be happy to do your shopping, post your letters for you, or do something in the house you can't manage. Other people will be able to keep you company sometimes, listen to you and share your worries and fears.

If you have to go into hospital and leave your house, pets or your garden, you can ask friends to help. If this is difficult, you could perhaps tell one friend what needs to be done, and ask them to organise things for you. You may find it hard to ask favours of people, but you will probably find that your friends are only too happy to be given specific things they can do for you.

Many of the organisations listed on pages 46–52 offer advice, information and support for people living on their own. Our cancer support service can give further information tailored to your needs. We have a factsheet about getting help with pet care when you are ill. Community, district and Macmillan nurses can also provide support and information about help at home (see page 35).

Emotional help

Counselling

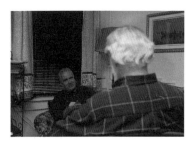

At times of stress and uncertainty some people find it helpful to talk to someone outside their immediate circle. Counsellors are trained to listen and help people to deal with difficult situations. They may be able to help you to find your own solutions to the problems you face. This can be very helpful, as cancer can affect many aspects of your life. Talking to someone who is supportive, and at the same time objective, can also help relatives.

Your GP or hospital doctor may be able to refer you to a counsellor. You may prefer to go to someone quite independent, away from where you are known. We can give you information about how to contact a counsellor in your area (see page 44). The Cancer Counselling Trust offers counselling to anyone affected by cancer (see page 49).

Groups

However supportive your family and friends, you may find it useful to spend some time with people who are sharing a similar experience to your own and coping with the ups and downs of their cancer.

There are now many support groups for people with cancer and their relatives. Most have been started by someone who felt the need to meet other people in a similar situation. Others are attached to hospitals. Some hospital cancer units or hospices have day centres or drop-in facilities for people who are at home.

Groups offer support and friendship of a particular kind. It can be reassuring to talk over your worries with someone who has been in a similar situation. It can also be very helpful to meet people who have lived with their cancer for a long time and who enjoy life.

We have information about support and self-help groups, and can give you details of organisations in your area.

Not everyone feels comfortable in a group and it is important that you take account of your own needs and preferences. You know yourself better than anyone else.

Things you might like to do for yourself

Complementary therapies

You may find meditation, visualisation, relaxation, aromatherapy or a combination of these techniques helpful. You can learn these from books or tapes, or there may be local classes. Your GP or practice nurse may know of these, or of someone who could teach you at home.

These are some of the techniques commonly used:

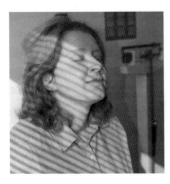

Relaxation involves learning to become aware of particular groups of muscles in your body and how to relax them. You can also use thoughts of space, heaviness or warmth in those areas. Once you have learnt how to do this, you can start using relaxation to reduce stress and tension.

Visualisation helps you to bring pleasant, relaxed pictures into your mind. Creating pictures and sounds in your mind that bring you pleasure can lessen stress and discomfort, and allow you to have a calmer state of mind.

We have a booklet called *Cancer and Complementary Therapies*, which gives information on complementary therapies and details of how to contact practitioners of these therapies.

Medicines

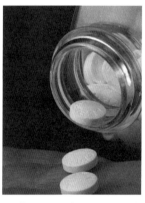

A lot of emotional distress can be reduced by the support of family, friends, self-help groups, counselling or some of the self-help techniques described above. However, sometimes your feelings of anxiety and depression start to interfere with your ability to deal with everything that is happening to you. In this case, your GP or hospital specialist may be able to help by prescribing antidepressants, anxiety-reducing drugs or sleeping pills. These can be very helpful in allowing you to cope with your situation.

We have a booklet called *The Emotional Effects of Cancer*, which can help you to deal with the feelings and emotions caused by advanced cancer.

Coping with day-to-day life

Coping with cancer that has spread or come back can involve an enormous amount of uncertainty. You may be worried about your treatment; pain or other symptoms; or not being able to do things for yourself, or to get around easily. You may be concerned about how you will be cared for as your cancer develops. You may have thoughts about death, people you would leave behind, or what happens after death.

Anxiety about the future is normal, especially when you have a serious illness that may focus your attention on your fears. There may be times when you feel that cancer is on your mind all the time, and you cannot spare any thoughts for anything else. But you do not have to cope with your fears on your own. There are a number of sources of help for you to turn to for practical advice, medical information, emotional support or spiritual comfort. You may find that, when some of your worries have been addressed, your mind will feel less burdened, and you will feel free to concentrate on living life the way you want to.

Setting your priorities

Some people with cancer say that they have a better appreciation of the ordinary things of life, such as family and friends, hobbies, a favourite book, picture or piece of music. Many people find their lives are more focused and they are less irritated by day-to-day problems.

Knowing that your illness may not be curable can give you an opportunity to decide what is important to you, and how you want to spend your time. You may have to give up some long-term plans, but you do not have to abandon all your ambitions. You may find that you now have the time to take up an activity that you have always been too busy to do before. Concentrating on what you can achieve and enjoy can give you pleasure and may help you to cope when you cannot meet other aims.

'The quality of life becomes more important than the quantity. I began to enjoy listening to music and, most of all, taking time to read.'

Talking to your doctor

Your worries about your cancer and treatment may be eased with information. Doctors may not be able to answer all your questions, but you have the right to ask about whatever you want to know.

Questions you may want to ask your doctor

- What are the options for treatment?
- How long will it be before I feel the benefit of any treatment?
- Can you give me some idea of how long I am likely to live?
- What help is available if my condition gets worse?
- Can I go on working? Should I try to negotiate shorter hours or part-time work?
- Will the illness affect my holiday/travelling plans?
- Will I need extra help in the house or with the children?
- Can I go on driving?

Physical frailty

You may find that you easily become very tired, and that your body is no longer as strong and reliable as it once was. This may be because of the cancer or because of the side effects of treatment. It may feel as though you have no strength and everything is more of an effort. It can be difficult to adjust if you can no longer drive or take part in sports, or have to walk more slowly than before. It will take time for you to get used to these changes and to accept having to rest, or the loss of activities that you once took for granted.

'When I ask my daughters over for a meal, I'm not really up to cooking it. They don't seem to mind – I buy the food and they cook it – but I feel I'm letting them down as I've always done the cooking.'

If your energy is limited, save it for the things you really want to do. Very often, re-organising your daily activities can be helpful – for example, by setting aside a time to rest every day. In addition, practical aids such as wheelchairs can be useful. You may feel that by using a walking stick, frame or wheelchair you are 'giving in' to your illness, but they can greatly improve your life by allowing you to move around more than you could do on your own.

We have a booklet, *Coping With Fatigue*, with tips on saving energy and coping with tiredness.

Being dependent

A very real fear for people with cancer is that they may lose their independence and dignity. Many people find the idea of being physically dependent on others deeply upsetting. It is often easier to accept help of an intimate kind (for example, being helped to wash, or go to the toilet) from a professional carer, than from your close family or friends. If you find this is the case, ask your GP or social worker to arrange help for you. Some of the organisations listed on pages 46–52 may also be able to provide services.

Even if you do need day-to-day care, you can still be independent in other ways and take the initiative in saying how you would like to be helped. For example, you could set a schedule for getting-up, washing and dressing, or organise a rota for other family members.

Looking after someone who is ill is a practical way for families and friends to show how much they care. If you can tell them what you need, and how they can best help you, there will be less room for misunderstanding and resentment if things do not go right all the time. You will also feel that your life is still your own.

While some people prefer to stay in their own homes in familiar surroundings, some may choose to move, perhaps because they live alone. In making this decision it may helpful to discuss with your family and friends where you would like to be looked after. You should be able to obtain support and information from your GP or social worker. Pages 34–40 discuss the different places where you can be looked after and the support available.

Controlling your symptoms

Pain

Not everyone with advanced cancer has pain, and for people who do get pain it can usually be well controlled. If you have pain that is disturbing you it needs to be treated, and it is important to let your doctor know. With modern painkillers you do not have to feel drowsy all the time to have good pain relief.

Non-drug treatments for pain can be used alone or as well as drug treatments. They include radiotherapy, nerve blocks, transcutaneous electrical nerve stimulation (TENS), acupuncture, hypnotherapy and relaxation techniques. Specialist pain clinics offer these methods of pain control, and your GP or cancer specialist can refer you to one of the clinics or to a symptom-control team.

Nausea and vomiting

Some people with advanced cancer have nausea and vomiting. This may be due to the type of cancer or may be a side effect of some medicines. You should let your doctor or nurse know if you have nausea or vomiting, as a lot can be done to relieve or control it. It can be helpful to avoid fatty and fried foods. Eating small meals and snacks, and taking small amounts of fizzy drinks, can also help to prevent nausea and vomiting. Our booklet, *Diet and Cancer*, has lots of suggestions for coping with eating problems and there is also a factsheet on controlling nausea and vomiting.

Other symptoms that may occur and which can be treated or relieved include:

- tiredness
- loss of appetite

- bowel or bladder problems

- breathlessness

- skin rashes

- sleep disturbances

- swollen ankles and legs.

The causes of pain and other symptoms, and treatments that may be used, are discussed in our booklets, *Controlling Cancer Pain* and *Controlling the Symptoms of Cancer*, which we can send to you.

Facing an uncertain future

'I still have not given up hope – my days are still bearable and I have survived to see my daughter marry. I only expected to see my son reach primary school, and now he is in his second year at comprehensive.'

One of the first questions anyone diagnosed with cancer is likely to have in their mind is 'Am I going to die?' This fear can become more intense if you are told that your cancer has spread or come back. For some people, cancer can become like any other chronic illness – something which causes problems from time to time, but which can be controlled. You may be able to lead a nearly normal life, even if the cancer is not curable.

Sometimes, though, the cancer develops and there may come a time when you realise that you will not recover. You may have decided that you do not want further treatment. Once again, emotions like fear, anger, guilt, sadness and disbelief may feel overwhelming. You may find that your mood swings between hope and despair.

There is no right or wrong way to face this situation. Each person has to try to deal with approaching death in their own way and at their own pace. Many people find a sense of peace and appear to be ready to 'let go' when the time comes.

People who are seriously ill, and the people close to them, will sometimes find themselves at a loss for words. But often simply being together is enough. A loving look, a hug or a squeeze of the hand can make words unnecessary. Tears are also very natural: you don't have to put on a brave face. If you try to hide your feelings, you and the people you love may not get the chance to say what is in your hearts.

You may find that your need for company and activity varies from day to day. Some people find they gradually need fewer people around them. As their energy fades, they may want to see only their closest friends, or their partner.

Some people do not want to be left alone at all during this time. When the person with cancer is being looked after at home, friends and relatives may be able to work out a rota so that there is always someone there. Hospitals and hospices can often arrange for a partner, relative or friend to stay overnight, every night.

Our booklet, *Dying With Cancer*, discusses what happens at the end of life and has details of the practical and emotional support available for the person who is dying and the people close to them.

Putting your affairs in order

It is natural to be concerned about how your possessions will be distributed after your death. It is a thoughtful and effective way of taking care of the people you love. It may also spare them painful decisions, bureaucratic hassles and even financial difficulty that might occur if you do not make your wishes clear. You may also find that once you have put your affairs in order, your mind is cleared of many concerns, leaving you free to concentrate on the present.

Making a will

Making a will ensures that you have control over your property. It makes sure that your loved ones, and people or issues that you care about, are looked after and that your wishes are carried out. If you die without making a will, the state decides who gets your possessions and it is unlikely that they will be shared out in the way you wish. You may find making a will a painful and upsetting thing to do; however, you may also gain a sense of satisfaction and relief at sorting out your affairs and knowing that you are safeguarding the future of your family and friends.

Making a will is not always as difficult or expensive as you might think, but it is a legal document and it should be properly prepared. It is advisable to go to a solicitor. A solicitor will know the precise wording to pass on your wishes and ensure they are carried out exactly as you want. If you do not use a solicitor, your will might not be clear and may cause delays and unnecessary legal expenses later on.

You can find a solicitor by asking a friend for a recommendation, or look in the Yellow Pages. Alternatively, phone the Law Society on 0870 606 6575 for England and Wales, or 0131 226

7411 for Scotland. It is best to telephone a few solicitors and get quotes before deciding which one is best for you. Solicitors will also sometimes make home visits.

If you have already made a will, you can update or alter it quite simply by adding a codicil. This is an extra instruction to your will which can be added at any stage, and alters it in any way you want. Again, it is helpful to prepare a list of the changes you want, then go to your solicitor, who can easily draw up the codicil for you.

Practical issues

Some practical things it might be helpful to do, include:

- Make a will (or update your will, if you have already made one).

- If you have children under 18, discuss arrangements for their future with your partner, and appoint guardians, in the event that you both die.

- List where you keep important documents (eg the title deeds of your house) and details of such things as your bank account, insurance premiums, etc.

- List the people who should be told when you die (eg your solicitor, if you have one; anyone who has been named as executor of your will; your employer; etc).

- Some people like to make plans for their own funeral, or discuss whether they would prefer cremation or burial.

It may be that there are everyday tasks you have always done that you should note down, so that there is some record of, for example, where you got the car serviced, how to turn the central heating boiler on, or how to use the washing machine.

Emotional affairs

In addition to dealing with your practical affairs, you may find that there are also emotional loose ends you want to tie up – for example, old friends you want to see, or perhaps quarrels you want to make up. If you want to contact someone you have not been in touch with for some time, you could try writing to or emailing them or phoning, telling them about your illness, and asking them to visit or get in touch with you. Approached with this sort of openness, old arguments can often be healed.

You may find yourself thinking a lot about the past, talking about joys, regrets and fears, going over events in your mind, perhaps going through old photo albums. You may want to visit places again, such as somewhere you used to live. If you are no longer able to get around by yourself, you can ask someone to take you or go with you.

You may also find yourself thinking about the future, and grieving for a time when you are no longer there. You may like to write letters to people who are dear to you, or perhaps prepare an audio or video tape, to be given to them after your death. Some people like to write down some of their family history for the next generation or to prepare a scrapbook for their children or grandchildren, perhaps getting the children to help.

These are sad things to do, but they can also be satisfying, as they give you a chance to think about the things that have happened to you, both good and bad – a kind of mental stocktake. They can also give you some amusement. The important thing is to do what feels right for you, when it feels right.

Family members or friends may feel that you are being morbid and gloomy and try to make you cheer up. Though this may be difficult for you, it is a sign of their love for you. It may be that they are not yet ready to accept what is happening. If you can, it may help to try and explain that you need time to yourself, to think and to feel sad.

Spiritual and religious issues

Some people find that they become more aware of religious or spiritual feelings during this time. People with a religious faith are often greatly supported by it during illness, but other people may also find that, perhaps for the first time in their lives, they need to think about and discuss spiritual issues. They may start thinking about whether there is a life after death. They may find comfort through prayer. Many people gain a great deal of support from knowing that other people are praying for them.

Even if you have not attended religious services regularly in the past, or you are not sure what you believe, you can still talk to a priest, rabbi or other religious leader. They are used to dealing with uncertainty and will not be shocked. They are not there to preach to you, but to comfort and help you find peace of mind.

If you are in hospital, you can ask for a visit from a hospital chaplain or appropriate religious or spiritual leader.

Who will look after me?

Your GP is the doctor who will have overall responsibility for your care. However, if you are having treatment such as chemotherapy or radiotherapy, you will usually go regularly to the hospital. At other times, the care you receive at home will be more important, and a number of people and organisations may be involved, working closely together.

Our booklet, *Caring for Someone With Advanced Cancer*, gives helpful information on the support available to you and the people caring for you.

Home care

Support is available for people being looked after at home, and help is also available for their carers. Unfortunately the availability of this support varies from one area of the UK to another. Your GP or social worker will probably be the best person to advise you on what is available in your area. The organisations listed on pages 46–52 will also be able to give you information.

The following is a brief guide to the people who are most likely to be involved in home care for someone with advanced cancer.

General practitioner (GP)

Overall responsibility for your care when you are being looked after at home lies with your GP. GPs are also responsible for prescribing any drugs you need, and for arranging admission to a hospital or hospice if necessary. They will assess your needs for nursing and medical care, and arrange the necessary help. Once the home care arrangements have been set up, you will probably see the community nurse more regularly than your GP.

Community nurses

Community or district nurses can pay regular visits. They offer nursing care services which may include changing dressings, giving medicines and supporting carers. They can also arrange practical aids such as pressure-relieving mattresses or commodes.

Specialist nurses (eg Macmillan)

These nurses are specialists in pain and symptom control, and in giving emotional support to patients and their families. They do not usually provide daily nursing care, but can visit you regularly to check on your symptoms and give advice. In some cases, they can teach you or your carer to give necessary medicines. They may be able to advise you about certain financial benefits you can apply for.

Macmillan nursing services are free. You can contact them through your GP or through their information line (page 51).

Marie Curie nurses

Marie Curie nurses are available in most parts of the UK and give a limited amount of day or night care in the home. The usual demand is for night nursing, so that the regular carer can get some rest. The services of Marie Curie nurses are free of charge and are usually arranged through the district nurse (see page 51).

Home care teams

These are usually based at a hospital or hospice, but work in the community with patients at home. The teams commonly include specialist nurses (often Macmillan nurses) who have had training in symptom control and emotional support. Sometimes the team includes a doctor who may share your care with your GP.

Psychologists

Psychologists may be able to help if you have anxiety or depression, and can look at ways to help you cope with everything that is going on. They can also help with relationship problems or if there has been a breakdown in communication within the family.

Occupational therapists

Occupational therapists, working in the community, are concerned with maintaining your comfort and independence at home. After an initial assessment, they may be able to arrange for aids such as toilet frames, handrails or a wheelchair to be delivered. They can also arrange for minor adaptations to your home, such as door-widening, or fixing safety rails in bathrooms. If you have difficulty dressing, they may be able to suggest and arrange alterations to clothing.

Physiotherapists

You can be put in touch with a physiotherapist by your GP or community nurse. They can help to keep you moving about, and also help to relieve pain, with treatment, massage and exercise programmes.

Help from social services

Care attendants/carers

Care attendants come into the home to give help of various kinds – either with jobs around the house such as cleaning, washing and cooking or just to sit with you, perhaps to give your carer some time off. They can also give some physical care such as washing and dressing. Some care attendant schemes provide someone to be there at night. Your local social services department, or Crossroads (address on page 47), will be able to tell you about schemes in your area.

Home helps

Home helps offer a variety of services including domestic help, cleaning, washing, cooking and shopping.

Home helps are available in some parts of the UK. Other districts, unfortunately, provide no service at all. Your local social services department, social worker, community nurse or GP will know the situation in your area. An assessment of your needs can be made through a social worker or care manager, or through hospital or community social services. You may have to contribute towards the cost of some services. Where no alternative exists, you can apply for a grant from Macmillan Cancer Support (see page 51).

Other sources of help

The Red Cross (main address on page 46) has a branch in every county and thousands of volunteers who can help you in many ways. These include shopping, posting letters and changing library books. They also lend equipment for nursing someone at home, such as wheelchairs and commodes, and provide an escort service to take people to hospital.

The Disabled Living Foundation (see page 47) runs an information service. It has specialist advisers on incontinence and clothing, and occupational therapists and physiotherapists can give personal advice on aids and equipment. Its showrooms have more than 2000 pieces of specialist equipment on display, from special cutlery to walking aids and wheelchairs. You can ask them for a catalogue.

In many areas there are volunteer schemes through which you can arrange for someone to visit your home, to provide company for you and a break for your carer. You can contact your local Community Volunteer Service or the Volunteer Bureau to find out what is available locally, and you could see if any information is displayed on notice boards in your GP's surgery, your local library, community centre or church.

Hospital and hospice care

If your illness develops, your doctor or nurse may suggest that you would be more comfortable being looked after in a hospital or hospice. This may only be for a short time so that your symptoms can be controlled, and you will then be able to go home again. Some hospitals have specialised units (palliative care units) which offer similar care to a hospice.

What is a hospice?

Hospices are places which specialise in symptom control, and also the care of people who are dying. The emphasis is on controlling pain and other symptoms, and supporting the person with cancer and their family. Hospices are smaller and quieter than hospitals and often work ut a gontler pace. Many offer bereavement support to relatives.

There are now more than 200 hospices in the UK. Many have home care teams and day centres for people living at home. Some are set up as part of the health service and others are funded by charity. They do not give long-term care. Care in a hospice is always free. Sometimes there may be a waiting list, but this is not usually longer than a few weeks.

You can find out more about your local hospice from your GP or by contacting the Hospice Information service (page 48).

Services offered by hospices

Some hospices work mainly through day centres, where people can go for one or two days a week. Often they have home care teams – doctors and nurses from the hospice visiting people in their own homes. Some hospices have beds for in-patients and these are often used for short stays, to get troublesome symptoms under control or to give carers a break and patients a change of scene. This is known as respite care.

Aren't they very depressing?

Many hospices are purpose-built, in pleasant grounds, and are designed to be attractive and comfortable. Many have kitchens, sitting rooms and accommodation for relatives. They also organise a range of activities for people who are well enough to take part.

It is normal to feel sad if you can no longer manage at home. You may also feel anxious, and worry about not being able to go home. These feelings may be eased by the benefits of staying in a hospice and being looked after by nurses and doctors who specialise in this sort of care. If you or your relatives are not sure about whether it is right for you, you can ask to visit first. Staff know that people often need to see for themselves, and will be happy to show you around and listen to your concerns.

Nursing homes

A residential home or private nursing home can be an alternative source of accommodation. They usually offer short-stay or respite care, but sometimes also offer long-stay care. Your GP, district nurse or social worker can arrange this for you. A fee is charged at private nursing homes and residential homes. Access to free care is sometimes possible, but is dependent on an assessment which is carried out by a social worker or care manager.

Availability of care varies from area to area and can take a while to organise. Lists of registered care homes, and details of registered nursing homes, are available from your local social services department and your area health authority. You can get information about finding a nursing home, and related issues, from the nursing home fees agency at www.nhfa.co.uk

Financial help and benefits

Illness nearly always involves unexpected expenses, and may reduce your income. Help is available from a number of sources and can sometimes be available at short notice.

Benefits

If you are **employed and unable to work**, your employer can pay you Statutory Sick Pay (SSP) for a maximum of 28 weeks.

If you are still unable to work after this period, you may be able to claim Incapacity Benefit. There are three rates of Incapacity Benefit: a short-term lower rate, a short-term higher rate and a long-term rate. You can claim the short-term higher rate of benefit from the Benefits Agency if you have paid the correct level of National Insurance contributions. If you are still unable to work after one year, you can claim long-term Incapacity Benefit.

If you are **self-employed** you are entitled to the same benefits as long as you have been paying the correct National Insurance contributions.

People who are **unemployed and unable to work** cannot claim Job Seeker's Allowance, but can apply to see if they qualify for the short-term lower rate of Incapacity Benefit. People who are not eligible for Incapacity Benefit because they have not paid the relevant National Insurance contributions may qualify for Income Support.

If you are **ill and not able to work**, remember to ask your GP for a medical certificate for the period of your illness. If you are in hospital, ask your doctor or nurse for a certificate to cover the time that you are an inpatient. This will be necessary if you need to claim a benefit. You may need to take a medical test to see if you are eligible to claim.

You may qualify for **Disability Living Allowance** (if you are under 65) or for Attendance Allowance (if you are over 65). Ask your local Social Security office for claim forms. There is a fast-track claim for people who may not live longer than 6 months. People who are claiming under this 'special rule' need to get their doctor to complete a form for either benefit. It is impossible to tell exactly how long someone may live and many people with advanced cancer may be entitled to this benefit, so it can be helpful to check with your doctor.

You may also be able to get **tax credits** from the Inland Revenue such as Child Tax Credit and Working Tax Credit. You can get information about these from a social worker, Citizens Advice Bureau, the Department for Work and Pensions, or the Tax credits Helpline 0845 300 3900.

The Benefits Agency has two booklets (IB1 and SD1) which outline all these benefits and others you may be entitled to. You can get a copy from your local Citizens Advice Bureau or Social Security office, where staff will also be able to advise you about the benefits you can claim. You will usually need to make an appointment. Their addresses and telephone numbers are in the phone book. You can also get information from the Benefit Enquiry Line on 0800 882200 or the Department for Work and Pensions website at www.dwp.gov.uk

The social worker at the hospital can give you advice on sources of financial help.

Direct Payments

If you have been assessed as having a need for social services, you may be entitled to get direct payments from your local authority. This means that you are given payments to organise social services yourself, rather than the local social services organising and paying for them for you. You can get information about direct payments from the Department of Health website at www.dh.gov.uk or from your local social security office.

Grants and Financial help

You may also be able to claim grants and benefits from other organisations or charities. Macmillan Cancer Supportgives grants to people with cancer and have a financial advice helpline (details on page 51). They produce a booklet called *Help With the Cost of Cancer*.

Your union or professional organisation, if you belong to one, may be able to give financial help or advice. For example, actors, bank employees, doctors, musicians, nurses, printers, social workers, members of the armed forces and teachers all have special funds which help with cash grants and sometimes holidays. Details are listed in *A Guide to Grants for Individuals in Need*, which is available in public libraries (see page 56 for details). It also gives details of all the trusts and organisations that provide financial support.

Viatical Settlements

Some specialist life assurance companies will buy life insurance policies for cash. This is known as a viatical settlement and can give you money at short notice. Care must be taken before selling an insurance policy, and we would recommend that you seek advice from an independent financial adviser.

In summary

We hope that this booklet helps to address some of the issues that may arise if you, or someone you know, is coping with advanced cancer. A lot of support is available, and helpful organisations, books, videos and websites are detailed on the following pages.

If you have further questions about any aspect of your situation, you can contact the nurses at Cancerbackup on 0808 800 1234.

Further information

Cancer Information and Support Service

The cancer information specialist nurses give information on all aspects of cancer and its treatment, and on the practical and emotional aspects of living with cancer.

Freephone: **0808 800 1234**
Lines are open Monday–Friday, 9am–8pm. An interpreting service is available for people whose first language is not English.

Calls to the Cancer Information and Support Service are confidential. Sometimes another member of our team may listen to a call for training purposes and to maintain quality.

You can also fax enquiries to **020 7696 9002** or email them to **info@cancerbackup.org**

or write to:

Cancerbackup, 3 Bath Place, Rivington Street, London, EC2A 3JR
Office: 020 7696 9003

Cancerbackup Scotland, Suite 2, 3rd Floor, Cranston House, 104–114 Argyle Street, Glasgow, G2 8BH
Office: 0141 223 7676 Freephone: 0808 800 1234

www.cancerbackup.org.uk

Cancerbackup's award-winning website includes the full text of all our publications, a database of support groups and other services for people affected by cancer.

Local centres

Cancerbackup also has local drop-in centres staffed by specialist cancer nurses:

- **Coventry**
  Cancerbackup Information
  Centre, Ground floor,
  University Hospital,
  Clifford Bridge Road,
  Coventry, CV2 2DX
  Tel: 02476 966 052

- **Ipswich**
  Cancer Information Centre,
  Woolverstone Wing,
  Ipswich Hospital, Heath Rd,
  Ipswich, IP4 5PD
  Tel: 01473 715 748

- **Jersey**
  Cancerbackup Jersey
  Gervais Les Gros Resource
  Centre, Mont les Vaux,
  St Aubin, Jersey, JE3 8AA
  Tel: 01534 498 235
  Freephone: 0800 7350 275

- **London**
  The Vicky Clement-Jones
  Cancerbackup Information
  Centre, King George V
  Building, St Bartholomew's
  Hospital, London, EC1A 7BE
  Tel: 020 7601 7936

- **London**
  Cancerbackup Information
  Centre, The London Clinic
  20 Devonshire Place,
  London, W1G 6BW
  Tel: 020 7616 7628

- **London**
  Cancerbackup Walk-in
  Information Centre,
  Charing Cross Hospital,
  Fulham Palace Road
  London, W6 8RF
  Tel: 020 8383 0171

- **Manchester**
  Cancer Information Centre,
  The Christie Hospital,
  Wilmslow Road,
  Withington
  Manchester, M20 4BX
  Tel: 0161 4468 100

- **Nottingham**
  Cancerbackup Information
  Centre, Oncology Block,
  Nottingham City Hospital,
  Hucknall Road,
  Nottingham, NG5 1PB
  Tel: 0115 8402 650

Other useful organisations

All contact details were correct at the time of going to press. Some may have changed. Current contact details can be checked on Cancerbackup's website at www.cancerbackup.org.uk/ Resourcessupport/Organisations

British Association for Counselling and Psychotherapy
BACP House, 35–37 Albert Street, Rugby, Warwickshire, CV21 2SG
Tel: 0870 4435 252
Fax: 0870 4435 161
Email: bacp@bacp.co.uk
Website: www.bacp.co.uk

BACP can refer people to a qualified local counsellor or organisation and can give basic information about therapy.

British Red Cross
44 Moorfields, London, EC2Y 9AL
Tel: 0870 1707 000.
Fax: 020 7562 2000
Email: information@redcross.org.uk
Website: www.redcross.org.uk

Services include: medical equipment loan, transport/escort service, home emergency personal care, home respite care, home from hospital and therapeutic care. Services can be accessed via the network of local Red Cross Branches throughout the UK.

Carers UK
Ruth Pitter House, 20–25 Glasshouse Yard, London, EC1A 4JT
CarersLine: 0808 808 7777 (Wednesday & Thursday, 10am–12pm & 2pm–4pm)
Tel: 020 7490 8818

Fax: 020 7490 8824
Minicom: 020 7251 8969
Email: info@ukcarers.org
Website: www.carersonline.org.uk

Offers information and support to professionals, relatives, and friends who are carers. Has 117 local and regional groups covering England, Northern Ireland, Scotland and Wales. Puts people in contact with carers' support groups in their area.

Crossroads – Caring for Carers
10 Regent Place, Rugby, Warwickshire, CV21 2PN
Tel: 0845 4500 350
Fax: 01788 565 498
Email: communications@crossroads.org.uk
Website: www.crossroads.org.uk

Provides practical respite care for carers, with over 200 schemes across England and Wales. Has sister organisations in Scotland and Northern Ireland.

Disability Alliance
Universal House, 88–94 Wentworth Street, London, E1 7SA
Tel (and minicom): 020 7247 8776 (Monday–Friday, 10am–4pm)
Fax: 020 7247 8765
Email: office.da@dial.pipex.com
Website: www.disabilityalliance.org

The leading authority on social security benefits and services for disabled people. Publishes a detailed handbook on disability rights and gives general information and personal advice.

Disabled Living Foundation
380–384 Harrow Road, London, W9 2HU
Helpline: 0845 1309 177 (weekdays, 10am–4pm)
Fax: 020 7266 292   Textphone: 020 7432 8009
Email: info@dlf.org.uk

Website: www.dlf.org.uk

Gives information and advice on products to assist independent living.

Family Welfare Trust

501–505 Kingsland Road, London, E8 4AU
Tel: 020 7254 6251
Fax: 020 7249 5443
Website: www.fwa.org.uk
Email: fwa.headoffice@fwa.org.uk

Offers a professional support and counselling service for families in distress and gives grants to people and families in need. Referral is by health or social care worker.

Hospice Information

Help the Hospices, Hospice House, 34 Britannia Street, London, WC1X 9JG
Tel: 0870 9033 903 (local rate)
Tel: 020 7520 8232 (Monday–Friday, 9am–5pm)
Email: info@hospiceinformation.info
Website: www.hospiceinformation.info

Offers an enquiry service, covering all aspects of hospice care, a website and a directory of hospice services in the UK and Eire.

National Association of Disablement Information and Advice Services (DIAL UK)

St Catherine's, Tickhill Road, Balby, Doncaster, South Yorkshire, DN4 8QN
Tel: 01302 310 123
Fax: 01302 310 404
Text Phone: 01302 310 123 (please use voice announcer)
Email: informationenquiries@dialuk.org.uk
Website: www.dialuk.info

The national organisation for the DIAL network of over 100

disability information and advice services. Groups are run by people with direct experience of disability. They give free, independent, impartial advice to disabled people, carers and professionals.

Relate
Herbert Grey College, Little Church Street, Rugby, Warwickshire, CV21 3AP
Appointments booking line: 0845 1304 016 (Monday–Friday 9am–5pm)
Tel: 01788 573 241
Fax: 01788 535 007
Email: enquiries@relate.org.uk
Website: www.relate.org.uk

Offers counselling, psychosexual therapy and educational services to couples wanting help with their relationship. Some centres cater for speakers of Asian or European languages as well as English. Local offices are listed in the phone book under Relate or marriage guidance.

General support and cancer organisations

Cancer Counselling Trust
1 Noel Road, London, N1 8HQ
Tel: 020 7704 1137
Email: support@cctrust.org.uk
Website: www.cctrust.org.uk

Qualified counsellors and psychotherapists offer free, confidential counselling to cancer patients, as well as couples or families affected by cancer. Face to face counselling is provided at the London office, and phone counselling is available for people unable to visit. Although the counselling is free, donations are welcomed if people are able to do so.

Citizens Advice Bureau (CAB)

For contact details for your nearest CAB, phone 020 7833 2181. Contact details will also be in your local phone book. Website: www.adviceguide.org.uk (Advice Guide)

An independent network that provides free, impartial information and advice about money, legal & other matters. Has offices around the UK. The website has up-to-date, comprehensive information on many topics, including the NHS. There are separate versions for each UK country, and are also available in English or several other languages.

Independent Financial Advisers Promotions Ltd (IFAP)

2nd floor, 117 Farringdon Road, London, EC1R 3BX
Consumer hotline: 0800 0853 250
Type talk: 0800 0830 196
Website: www.ifap.org.uk
Email: contact@ifap.org.uk

IFAP aims to help people search for details of local member independent financial advisers via the consumer hotline and online searches via www.unbiased.co.uk and www.fsa.gov.uk/consumer

Irish Cancer Society

43–45 Northumberland Road, Dublin 4, Ireland
Cancer Helpline: 1800 200 700
Action Breast Cancer (ABC) Helpline: 1800 309 040
Email: helpline@irishcancer.ie
Website: www.cancer.ie

The national charity dedicated to preventing cancer, saving lives from cancer and improving the quality of life of people in Ireland living with cancer through patient care, research and education.

Macmillan Cancer Support

89 Albert Embankment, London, SE1 7UQ
Macmillan CancerLine: 0808 8082 020

Macmillan Benefit Helpline: 0808 8010 304
Email: cancerline@macmillan.org.uk
Website: www.macmillan.org.uk

Provides specialist advice and support through Macmillan nurses and doctors, and financial advice and grants for people with cancer and their families.

Marie Curie Cancer Care
89 Albert Embankment, London, SE1 7TP
Tel: 020 7599 7777
Email: info@mariecurie.org.uk
Website: www.mariecurie.org.uk

Runs a number of hospice centres for cancer patients throughout the UK, and a community nursing service, which works in conjunction with the district nursing service to support cancer patients and their carers in their homes.

Personal Finance Society
20 Aldermanbury, London, EC2V 7HY
Tel: 020 8530 0852
Fax: 020 7796 3882
Email: customer.serv@thepfs.org
Website: www.thepfs.org

The Personal Finance Society is the UK's largest professional body for individual financial advisers (and those in related roles). It is part of the Chartered Insurance Institute.

Tak Tent Cancer Support – Scotland
Flat 5, 30 Shelley Court, Gartnavel Complex, Glasgow, G12 0YN
Tel: 0141 2110 122
Email: tak.tent@care4free.net
Website: www.taktent.org.uk

Offers information, support, education and care for cancer patients, families, friends and professionals. Has a network of support groups throughout Scotland and a drop-in resource and information centre at the above address.

Tenovus Cancer Information Centre
Velindre Hospital, Whitchurch, Cardiff, CF14 2TL
Freephone helpline: 0808 8081 010 (Monday–Friday, 09.00–16.30)
Tel: 029 2019 6100
Email: tcic@tenovus.com
Website: www.tenovus.com

Provides an information service on all aspects of cancer, and emotional support for cancer patients and their families.

The Ulster Cancer Foundation
40–42 Eglantine Avenue, Belfast, BT9 6DX
Freephone helpline: 0800 7833 339
Tel: 028 9066 3281
Email: info@ulstercancer.org
Website: www.ulstercancer.org

Provides a cancer information helpline, patients' resource and information centre, support groups and a range of booklets for patients and relatives.

Helpful books

Beyond Fear
Dorothy Rowe
Harper Collins, 2002
ISBN 0-007119-24-0   £12.99

Written by a psychologist, this book argues that we all fear loss, bereavement, old age, rejection, failure, and, most of all, death. And that, we deny our fear in order not to be thought weak, which can lead to physical illness, or to mental problems. It discusses how to have the courage to face and work with fear.

The Complete Guide To Relieving Cancer Pain And Suffering
Richard B Patt
Oxford University Press, 2004
ISBN 0-195135-01-6   £21.50

This book helps cancer patients, their carers and families make informed decisions about living with cancer, and the range of treatments available. Although some sections are specific to the US, it is still useful for people in the UK.

Life Choices, Life Changes: Develop Your Personal Vision With Image Work (New Ed.)
Dina Glouberman
Hodder & Stoughton, 2004
ISBN 0-340826-77-0   £8.99

A discussion about using imagery and visualisation to develop and improve your life, confidence and situation.

The New Natural Death Handbook (3rd Ed.)
Nicholas Albery & Stephanie Wienrich (eds.)
The Natural Death Centre, 2000
ISBN 0-712605-76-2   £10.99

Covers many topics relating to 'green' or natural funerals, such as a good funeral guide to the best funeral directors, and woodland burial grounds. Also covers preparing for dying and caring for a dying person at home, drawing up a will and advance funeral wishes (living wills), and memory boxes (available from Barnardos).

Jewish Perspectives On Illness And Healing
Ellen Levine
Rutledge Books
ISBN: 1-582441-34-0   £8.37

A look at Jewish perspectives on illness and healing.

The Road Less Traveled: A New Psychology Of Love, Traditional Values And Spiritual Growth
M Scott Peck
Rider, 2003
ISBN 0-712661-15-8   £7.99

Written by a psychologist, gives gentle guidance on dealing with emotional pain and developing contentment and confidence.

Mind Of Clear Light: Advice On Dying And Living Well
His Holiness Dalai Lama
Publisher: Pocket Books, 2004
ISBN: 0-743244-69-9

Discusses how to use life as a preparation for death, and approach death as a natural part of life. Written in a warm, sensitive style with humour.

Meetings At The Edge: Dialogues With The Grieving And The Dying, The Healing And The Healed
Stephen Levine
Gateway, 2002
ISBN 0-717133-41-9   £10.99

Written by a man with extensive experience of dealing with

people who face death. Sensitively explores all aspects of death and the feelings and emotions people may have.

Walking Toward The Light: Accepting Cancer With Faith And Resolve
Robert Bruce
Publisher: iUniverse.com, 2005
ISBN: 0-595340-37-7   £7.61

A detailed account of the author's struggle to understand his wife's cancer diagnosis, and his eventual acceptance of her inevitable death. Advises how to overcome the challenges that arise when a relative or friend is diagnosed with cancer.

General books

Cancer at your Fingertips (3rd ed)
Val Speechley and Maxine Rosenfield
Class Publishing, 2001
ISBN: 1-859590-36-5   £14.99

Written by two experts in the field, this manual answers over 450 questions that people most commonly ask about cancer. It deals thoroughly with common concerns regarding the causes of cancer, the treatment options available and ways of living with – and after – treatment for cancer.

Challenging Cancer: Fighting Back, Taking Control, Finding Options (2nd ed)
Maurice Slevin and Nina Kfir
Class Publishing, 2002
ISBN: 1-859590-68-3   £14.99

Written by a cancer specialist and a psychotherapist, this book aims to help people make sense of a cancer diagnosis to regain control of their lives. Also includes a section on Vicky Clement-Jones the founder of Cancerbackup.

A Guide to Grants for Individuals in Need 2004/2005
Alan French, Dave Griffiths and Emma Jepson
Directory of Social Change, 2004
ISBN: 1-903991-52-8   £29.95

A directory of over 2000 charities and trusts that provide financial help to people in need. Also lists each organisation's criteria and how to apply.

Help with the Cost of Cancer: a Guide to Benefits and Financial Help for People Affected by Cancer
Macmillan Cancer Support, 2004

This free booklet provides information about all of the different kinds of financial help available for people with cancer. To order call Macmillan Cancerline on 0808 808 2020, email cancerline@macmillan.org.uk or download a copy from www.macmillan.org.uk

Taking Control of Cancer
Beverley Van Der Molen
Class Publishing, 2003
ISBN: 1-859590-91-8   £14.95

A useful and supportive book, which is helpful for people who have been diagnosed with any type of cancer, or for their family and friends.

Understanding Cancer
Gareth Rees
Family Doctor Publications, 2002
ISBN: 1-898205-51-5   £3.50

Clearly written and well-illustrated. Gives information on what cancer is, how the diagnosis is made and treatments. Diagnostic tests are explained and illustrated. Also touches briefly on symptom control, clinical trials and complementary treatments.

Useful websites

A lot of information about cancer is available on the internet. Some websites are excellent; others have misleading or out-of-date information. The sites listed below are considered by doctors to contain accurate information and are regularly updated.

www.cancerbackup.org.uk (Cancerbackup)

- Contains over 4500 pages of accurate, up-to-date information on all aspects of cancer and a searchable database of other organisations.

- Allows you to send questions to specialist cancer nurses by email and has a question-and-answer section.

- Contains all Cancerbackup's 70+ booklets and 260+ factsheets included in full.

- Recommends further reading.

- Provides discussion for health professionals and others on cancer issues.

- Has a search engine for cancer research clinical trials available to cancer patients in the UK and Europe

- Offers links to recommended cancer websites around the world.

www.cancerhelp.org.uk (Cancer Research UK)
Contains patient information on all types of cancer and has a cancer research clinical trials database.

www.nhsdirect.nhs.uk (NHS Direct Online)

www.nhsdirect.wales.nhs.uk (NHS Direct Wales)

www.nhs24.com (NHS 24 in Scotland)

NHS health information sites for England, Scotland and Wales – covers all aspects of health, illness and treatments.

www.nci.nih.gov (National Cancer Institute – National Institute of Health – USA)

Contains patient information on all types of cancer and treatments.

www.carers.gov.uk

A Department of Health website providing details of the services and benefits affecting carers.

www.cancer.gov/cancertopics/advancedcancer

An online version of a booklet produced by the US National Cancer Institute. Gives comprehensive information on cancer and treatments.

www.dipex.org (Database of individual patient experiences)

Contains information about some cancers and has video and audio clips of people talking about their experiences of cancer and its treatments. Also contains discussion of the physical, social and psychological effects of cancer.

Cancerbackup editorial policy

Cancerbackup's policy is to provide up-to-date and accurate information about cancer and its treatments, in line with accepted national and international guidelines. Where no such guidelines exist, our information is based on scientific evidence such as data from published clinical trials, or combined analyses of trials. Where such evidence is not available, our information is based on a consensus view of experts. Each Cancerbackup publication is regularly reviewed and updated by cancer doctors, specialist nurses, other relevant health professionals and patients. The medical information is approved by a member of Cancerbackup's Clinical Advisory Board and the Medical Editor.

All Cancerbackup's booklets that describe treatments are produced to meet the criteria of the Discern Index, a nationally recognised measure of health information quality. Where trusts have used Cancerbackup's booklets in evidence to support their good practice, it has helped them to achieve compliance with the standards of the Clinical Negligence Scheme for Trusts. The content of Cancerbackup publications is independent of sponsorship.

Cancerbackup Clinical Advisory Board

Chair: Dr Tim Eisen

Ms Deborah Bernardes; Dr Peter Blake; Ms May Bullen; Ms Debbie Coats; Ms Christine Clarke; Professor Hugh Coakham; Professor Karen Cox; Ms Stephanie Davies; Mr Mike Dixon; Professor Edzard Ernst; Mr John Fielding; Ms Judy Gunn; Professor Rajnish Gupta; Dr Peter Harvey; Ms Amelia Lee; Professor David Luesley; Dr James Mackay; Ms Pauline McCulloch; Ms Peggotty Moore; Professor Gareth Morgan; Professor Peter Mortimer; Dr Ann Naysmith; Dr Chris Parker ; Dr Terry Priestman; Dr Clare Shaw; Dr Amen Sibtain; Dr Maurice Slevin; Mr Andrew Stanley; Ms Sandra Tang; Dr Andrew Webb; Dr Jeremy Whelan; Ms Val Young

This booklet has been produced in accordance with the following sources and guidelines:

- *Manual of Cancer Services Standards*. NHS Executive, 2001.

- *Palliative Cancer Care Guidelines*. Scottish Partnership Agency for Palliative and Cancer Care, 1994.

- *Supportive and Palliative Care for People with Cancer*. National Institute of Clinical Excellence (NICE), 2005.

- *Oxford Textbook of Palliative Medicine*. Eds: Derek Doyle, et al. Oxford University Press, 1999.

- *Symptom Management in Advanced Cancer*. Robert Twycross. Radcliffe Medical Press, 2001.

You can access up-to-date guidelines in the health professional section of Cancerbackup's website: www.cancerbackup.org.uk

Questions you might like to ask your doctor or nurse

You can fill this in before you see the doctor or nurse, and then use it to remind yourself of the questions you want to ask, and the answers you receive.

1. ....

Answer ....

....

2. ....

Answer ....

....

3. ....

Answer ....

....

4. ....

Answer ....

....

5. ....

Answer ....

....

6. ....

Answer ....

....